HERBAL TEA GARDENING FOR BEGINNERS

The comprehensive guide on how to grow, care, harvest and brew tea at home

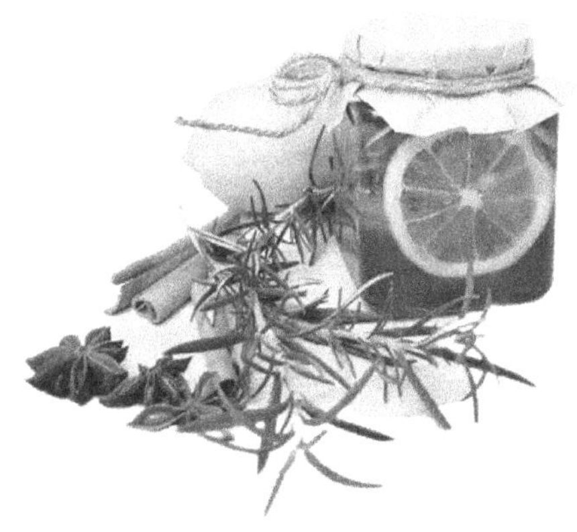

Larry Pat

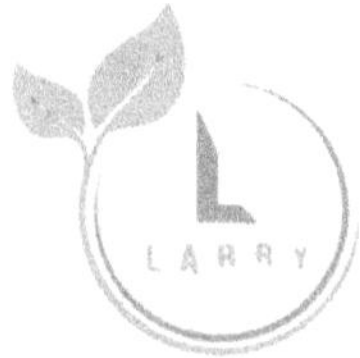

TABLE OF CONTENT

INTRODUCTION

Welcome to the world of cultivating your own tea garden! Embark on the journey of discovering the finest herbs to nurture for a charming herbal tea haven. Ideal for windowsills or garden beds, growing your own herbs not only ensures a more robust and aromatic tea but also brings a myriad of healing benefits, ranging from soothing anxieties to enhancing sleep.

Immerse yourself in this simple and delightful way to connect with nature!
If you've ever encountered bland and uninspiring tea, chances are it was either the herbs or the brewing

method—both challenges with straightforward solutions! Let's delve into the realm of herbs.

Reasons to Cultivate a Tea Garden

1. Delectable Taste: When creating an herb garden specifically for tea, opt for homegrown herbs like mint, lemon balm, and chamomile. These varieties surpass store-bought options, often grown in less flavorful hothouses.

2. Healing Potency: Many herbs boast natural healing properties. Lemon balm, mint, and chamomile, for instance, have been historically utilized to alleviate stress and promote restful sleep. The roots of herbal medicine trace back thousands of years to the

Sumerians, who employed tea infusions to address inflammation and congestion. Herbal remedies have been a cornerstone in apothecaries, marking the genesis of modern medicine. Beyond medicinal uses, the experience of cultivating and sipping your own herbal tea is profoundly nurturing.

3. Ease of Cultivation: Creating a tea garden is remarkably simple! A modest space is all you need to grow herbs for steeping tea. Whether in a small garden bed, on a balcony, in containers, or on a windowsill, nearly all "tea plants" flourish across North America. These hardy perennials can withstand temperatures as low as -20°F.

4. Enjoyable and Relaxing: Growing a variety of herbs opens the door to blending different herbal teas and experimenting with flavors. Picture a blend of chamomile, lemon balm, and lavender—pure bliss! The delightful fragrances emitted by various herbs add an extra layer of pleasure. Moreover, your herbs can be utilized in myriad ways, from enhancing kitchen dishes to crafting herbal vinegars, soaps, bath soaks, and healing tinctures.

CHAPTER 1: ESSENTIAL TOOLS AND EQUIPMENT

BASIC GARDENING TOOLS

1. Trowel and Hand Fork

In your gardening journey, think of the trowel and hand fork as your dynamic duo for hands-on tasks. The trowel, with its flat, scoop-like blade, is perfect for digging small holes, transplanting seedlings, or breaking up soil. The hand fork, with its sturdy prongs, becomes your go-to for weeding and aerating soil. Look for ergonomically designed tools to ensure comfort during extended use.

2. Pruners and Shears

Pruning is a gardening art, and pruners and shears are your brush and palette. Pruners, designed for precision, are excellent for cutting stems and branches, promoting plant health. Shears come into play for shaping and trimming larger sections. Regular pruning encourages robust growth and helps maintain your herbs' desired shape.

3. Garden Gloves

Your hands are your most valuable tools, so protect them with reliable garden gloves. These not only shield you from dirt and thorns but also provide a comfortable grip. Opt for breathable, waterproof gloves to keep your hands dry and comfortable during various gardening tasks.

4. Watering Can or Hose

Water, the lifeblood of your herb garden, requires a reliable delivery system. A watering can or hose is your conduit for hydration. The gentle flow of a watering can ensure even distribution to the plant's base, while a hose provides versatility and convenience. Adequate watering is the key to preventing both drought stress and waterlogged roots.

5. Garden Knife or Scissors

Harvesting herbs is a satisfying culmination of your gardening efforts. A sharp garden knife or scissors is your harvesting companion, ensuring clean cuts without causing unnecessary stress to the plants. Harvesting correctly promotes continuous growth and enhances the flavor of your culinary herbs.

SOIL AND POTTING MIXTURES

Understanding Soil Types

Your herb garden's foundation lies in the soil beneath. Understand the three primary soil types: loamy, sandy, and clay. Loamy soil strikes the perfect balance, offering good drainage and fertility. Sandy soil allows for quick drainage, while clay soil retains moisture. Identify your soil type to tailor your gardening practices accordingly.

Importance of Good Drainage

Well-draining soil is your herbs' lifeline. It prevents water from stagnating around the roots, reducing the risk of root rot and other water-related issues. Enhance drainage by incorporating organic matter, such as compost, into your soil. Aim for soil that is crumbly and loose, allowing water to move freely.

Organic vs. Inorganic Soil Amendments

Choose your soil amendments wisely. Organic options, like compost and well-rotted manure, enrich the soil with essential nutrients and improve its structure. Inorganic additives, such as perlite and vermiculite, enhance aeration and drainage. Strike a balance that aligns with your gardening philosophy and the needs of your herbs.

Creating Your Own Potting Mix

Crafting a customized potting mix is akin to creating a tailored wardrobe for your herbs. Combine components like peat moss, perlite, and compost to create a well-balanced mix. Adjust proportions based on the specific requirements of your herbs, ensuring they have the ideal environment to thrive.

CONTAINERS AND PLANTERS

Choosing the Right Containers

Containers are the homes for your potted herbs, so choose wisely. Consider the size and growth habits of your herbs when selecting containers. Opt for materials like terracotta, which breathes and prevents waterlogging, or plastic for its lightweight and durable nature. Ensure containers have drainage holes to prevent water accumulation.

Container Materials and Their Pros/Cons

Dive deeper into the world of container materials. Terracotta, with its porous nature, allows for air exchange, but it can dry out quickly. Plastic containers are lightweight and retain moisture but may lack breathability. Wooden containers add a touch of natural aesthetics but require proper sealing to resist decay. Is good to understand the pros and cons to make informed decisions.

Size and Placement of Containers

Container size matters, influencing the health and growth of your herbs. Larger containers provide more room for root development, reducing the frequency of watering. Consider the mature size of your herbs and group compatible ones together. Pay attention to placement, ensuring your containers receive adequate sunlight and are sheltered from harsh weather conditions.

Vertical Gardening Options

Expand your gardening horizons by going vertical. Utilize trellises, hanging planters, and wall-mounted containers to maximize space and add visual interest to your herb garden. Vertical gardening is not just a space-saving technique; it's an artistic way to showcase your herbs. Experiment with different arrangements to create a vibrant and dynamic herb display.

CHAPTER 2: SELECTING HERBS FOR YOUR GARDEN

When it comes to herb selection, your choices are vast and varied. This chapter will guide you through the delightful process of choosing herbs for your garden, covering popular culinary herbs, medicinal herbs suitable for beginners, and aromatic herbs that add a fragrant touch to your green haven.

POPULAR CULINARY HERBS

Basil (Ocimum basilicum)

Basil is a kitchen favorite, known for its distinct aroma and versatile culinary applications. Whether you're making a classic pesto or enhancing the flavor of tomato dishes, basil is a must-have herb. There are various varieties, including sweet basil, Thai basil, and lemon basil, each offering unique flavors to elevate your cooking.

Rosemary (Rosmarinus officinalis)

With needle-like leaves and a woody fragrance, rosemary is a robust herb that pairs well with roasted meats and vegetables. Its resilience makes it suitable for both outdoor and indoor gardens. Consider trailing or upright varieties to suit your gardening preferences.

Parsley (Petroselinum crispum)

Parsley adds a fresh, vibrant touch to dishes and is a staple in many cuisines.

With curly and flat-leaf varieties, parsley is rich in vitamins and minerals. It's an excellent garnish and a key ingredient in herb blends like fine herbes.

Cilantro (Coriandrum sativum)

Cilantro brings a burst of citrusy flavor to your dishes, making it a key player in salsas, curries, and salads. Be mindful that cilantro has a relatively short growing season, so stagger your plantings for a continuous harvest.

Chives (Allium schoenoprasum)

These mild, onion-flavored herbs are perfect for snipping into salads, soups, and omelets. Chives produce lovely lavender blossoms that are not only edible but also attract beneficial pollinators to your garden.

MEDICINAL HERBS FOR BEGINNERS

Lavender (Lavandula spp.):

Beyond its enchanting fragrance, lavender has calming properties, making it a popular choice for herbal remedies. Considered beginner-friendly, lavender is versatile—use it in sachets, teas, or infused oils for both its aromatic and therapeutic benefits.

Calendula (Calendula officinalis)

Known for its bright orange and yellow flowers, calendula is not just visually appealing; it also possesses medicinal properties. Calendula-infused oils can be used topically to soothe skin irritations and promote healing.

Echinacea (Echinacea purpurea)

Boost your immune system with the vibrant purple flowers of echinacea. This medicinal herb is renowned for its ability to help fend off colds and respiratory infections. It's a resilient perennial that adds both beauty and functionality to your garden.

Peppermint (Mentha × piperita)

Peppermint isn't just for tea; it's a digestive aid and can be used to alleviate headaches. Plant it in containers to prevent its rapid spread, and enjoy its fresh, invigorating aroma and taste.

Lemon Balm (Melissa officinalis)

A member of the mint family, lemon balm is prized for its lemony fragrance and calming properties. It's an excellent choice for herbal teas and can be used to support relaxation and ease stress.

AROMATIC HERBS FOR FRAGRANCE

Sage (Salvia officinalis)

Sage, with its velvety leaves and earthy aroma, is not only a culinary herb but also a delightful addition to your aromatic herb collection. Inhaling its scent is believed to promote mental clarity and relaxation.

Thyme (Thymus vulgaris)

Thyme's tiny leaves pack a powerful fragrance. This herb is a classic in culinary applications, but its aromatic qualities extend to providing a pleasant atmosphere in your garden. Consider varieties like lemon thyme for an extra aromatic punch.

Mint (Mentha spp.)

Mint varieties, such as spearmint and peppermint, offer invigorating scents. Plant them strategically to enjoy the refreshing aroma as you brush by. Keep in mind that mint can be vigorous, so it's often best grown in containers to control its spread.

Lemongrass (Cymbopogon citratus)

Known for its citrusy fragrance, lemongrass is a versatile herb used in both culinary and aromatic applications. Its tall, slender stalks add an exotic touch to your garden, and you can harvest them for teas or Asian-inspired dishes.

Lavender (Lavandula spp.)

Repeated from the medicinal herbs section, lavender earns a dual spot for its exceptional fragrance. Plant lavender strategically to enjoy its calming scent in your garden and harvest its blooms for various uses, from sachets to infused oils.

CHAPTER 3: STARTING HERBS FROM SEEDS AND SEEDLINGS

Embarking on the journey of growing herbs from seeds is a rewarding experience that allows you to witness the entire life cycle of your plants. This chapter guides you through the basics of seed starting, the delicate process of transplanting seedlings, and the art of propagating herbs to expand your garden.

SEED STARTING BASICS

Selecting Quality Seeds

Begin your herb-growing adventure by choosing high-quality seeds from reputable sources. Research on seeds that are fresh, viable, and suited to your climate. Consider heirloom varieties for a diverse and unique herb garden.

Choosing Seed Starting Containers

Opt for containers that provide good drainage and are suitable for seed starting. Use seed trays, peat pots, or recycled containers with drainage holes to prevent waterlogged soil and ensure healthy seedlings.

Sowing Depth and Timing

Different herbs have varying seed requirements, so pay attention to recommended sowing depths. Start seeds indoors according to your region's frost dates, ensuring that seedlings are robust and ready for transplanting when the outdoor growing season begins.

Ideal Germination Conditions

Create an optimal environment for germination by maintaining consistent moisture and warmth. Use a seed starting mix, keep the soil consistently moist but not waterlogged, and provide adequate warmth through heat mats or a warm indoor location.

TRANSPLANTING SEEDLINGS

Hardening Off Seedlings

Before transplanting seedlings into the garden, gradually acclimate them to outdoor conditions through a process known as hardening off. Expose seedlings to increasing amounts of sunlight and outdoor temperatures over several days to prevent shock.

Choosing the Right Time

Transplant seedlings when they have developed a strong root system and have at least two sets of true leaves. Ensure the risk of frost has passed, and the soil has warmed sufficiently for optimal growth.

Digging and Planting

Create a hole in the garden soil that accommodates the size of the seedling's root ball. Gently remove seedlings from their containers, taking care not to disturb the roots. Place each seedling in its designated hole, backfill with soil, and water thoroughly.

Spacing and Arrangement

Consider the mature size of your herbs when spacing seedlings in the garden. Adequate spacing ensures proper air circulation and prevents overcrowding, reducing the risk of diseases. Plan the arrangement to create an aesthetically pleasing and functional garden design.

PROPAGATING HERBS

Methods of Propagation

Herbs can be propagated through various methods, including division, cuttings, and layering. Learn about each technique to expand your herb garden and create new plants from existing ones.

Dividing Mature Plants

Many herbs, such as chives and mint, benefit from division. Carefully lift mature plants, separate them into smaller sections, and replant each division. This not only creates new plants but also revitalizes the original plant.

Taking Herb Cuttings

Propagation through cuttings involves taking a portion of a healthy stem, usually with a node, and encouraging it to root. This method is suitable for herbs like rosemary, lavender, and basil. Ensure your cutting has a few sets of leaves and remove any excess foliage to reduce stress on the plant.

Layering for New Growth

Layering is a technique where a portion of a healthy stem is bent to the ground, covered with soil, and encouraged to root. Once roots develop, the new plant can be separated and replanted. This method is effective for herbs like thyme and oregano.

CHAPTER 4: CARING FOR YOUR HERB GARDEN

Now that your herb garden is planted and thriving, it's time to delve into the essential aspects of care. This chapter focuses on providing your herbs with the attention they need to flourish, covering watering and drainage, soil amendments and fertilizing, and the art of pruning and harvesting.

WATERING AND DRAINAGE

Understanding Watering Needs

Herbs have varying water requirements, and understanding these needs is crucial for their overall health. While some herbs prefer consistently moist soil, others thrive in drier conditions. Pay attention to signs of overwatering or underwatering, such as wilting or yellowing leaves.

Consistent Moisture vs. Drying Out

Strike a balance between consistent moisture and allowing the soil to dry out slightly between waterings. Overly saturated soil can lead to root rot, while too little water can stress the plants. Adjust your watering schedule based on the specific needs of each herb and the prevailing weather conditions.

Watering Methods

Consider the watering method based on the herb's preferences and the garden layout. Use a gentle watering can for precision or a soaker hose for even distribution. Aim to water the base of the plants to minimize moisture on the foliage, reducing the risk of fungal diseases.

Improving Drainage

Ensure proper drainage to prevent waterlogged soil. If your garden soil retains water excessively, amend it with organic matter like compost or perlite to improve drainage. Elevating containers on bricks or adding a layer of gravel at the bottom helps excess water drain away efficiently.

SOIL AMENDMENTS AND FERTILIZING

Regular Soil Testing

Perform regular soil tests to assess the nutrient levels in your garden soil. This helps you make informed decisions about the type and amount of amendments needed. Soil tests are especially beneficial at the beginning of each growing season.

Organic Soil Amendments

Incorporate organic amendments like compost, well-rotted manure, or worm castings to enrich the soil with essential nutrients. These additions not only provide a nutrient boost but also enhance soil structure and support beneficial microbial activity.

Balanced Fertilization

Choose a balanced fertilizer or one specifically formulated for herbs to ensure your plants receive the necessary nutrients. Follow recommended application rates, and avoid over-fertilizing, as this can lead to nutrient imbalances and potentially harm your herbs.

Mulching for Nutrient Retention

Mulch serves as a protective layer, conserving soil moisture and suppressing weeds. Organic mulches, such as straw or shredded leaves, also break down over time, contributing valuable nutrients to the soil.

PRUNING AND HARVESTING
Promoting Healthy Growth Through Pruning

Pruning is a fundamental aspect of herb care, promoting bushier, more robust growth. Regularly pinch back the tips of your herbs, especially those with tender growth, to encourage branching. Remove dead or yellowing leaves to maintain plant vigor.

Harvesting Best Practices

Harvest herbs at the peak of their flavor and aroma. Snip or cut stems just above a leaf node to encourage new growth.

Avoid harvesting more than one-third of the plant at a time to ensure it continues to thrive.

Morning is often the best time to harvest when essential oils are most concentrated.

Drying and Storing Herbs

Drying herbs is an excellent way to preserve their flavors for later use. Harvest herbs on a dry day, tie them in bundles, and hang them in a cool, well-ventilated area. Once dry, store the herbs in airtight containers away from direct sunlight.

CHAPTER 5: COMMON PESTS AND DISEASES

As your herb garden flourishes, it becomes essential to safeguard your plants from potential threats. This chapter addresses the identification and prevention of common pests, explores natural pest control methods, and provides insights into recognizing and managing common diseases that may affect your precious herbs.

IDENTIFYING AND PREVENTING PESTS

Vigilance and Observation

Maintaining a vigilant eye on your herb garden is the first step in identifying pests. Regularly inspect the leaves, stems, and undersides of your plants for signs of damage, discoloration, or the presence of insects.

Common Herb Pests

Familiarize yourself with common herb pests such as aphids, spider mites, and caterpillars. Learn to recognize their distinctive damage patterns, whether it's stippling on leaves, curled foliage, or visible pests themselves.

Companion Planting for Pest Prevention

Implement companion planting strategies to naturally deter pests. Certain herbs, like basil and mint, have repellent properties that can protect neighboring plants. Integrate pest-resistant plants strategically throughout your garden to create a natural barrier against unwelcome visitors.

Healthy Soil, Healthy Plants

Maintain the health of your herbs by ensuring optimal soil conditions. Healthy plants are more resilient to pest infestations. Amend soil with organic matter, follow proper watering practices, and avoid over-fertilizing, which can attract certain pests

Natural Pest Control Methods

Beneficial Insects

Encourage the presence of beneficial insects, such as ladybugs, lacewings, and predatory beetles, which feed on common herb pests. Plant flowers like marigolds and calendula to attract these natural predators to your garden.

Neem Oil and Insecticidal Soap

Utilize natural remedies like neem oil and insecticidal soap to control pests. Neem oil disrupts the life cycle of many insects and acts as a repellent, while insecticidal soap suffocates soft-bodied pests like aphids. Apply these treatments sparingly and follow package instructions.

Homemade Pest Sprays

Create homemade pest sprays using ingredients like garlic, chili peppers, and soapy water. These concoctions can be effective in deterring pests and are safe for your herbs. Experiment with different recipes to find what works best for your specific pest challenges.

RECOGNIZING COMMON DISEASES

Fungal Diseases

Be on the lookout for common fungal diseases, such as powdery mildew and downy mildew, which can affect herb plants. Provide adequate spacing between plants to promote air circulation, and avoid overhead watering to minimize moisture on foliage.

Bacterial Infections

Bacterial infections, like bacterial leaf spot and bacterial wilt, can impact herb crops. Practice proper sanitation by removing and disposing of infected plant material promptly. Copper-based fungicides may help manage bacterial diseases.

Viral Infections

Viral infections can manifest as mottled or distorted foliage. Unfortunately, there are no direct cures for viral diseases. Prevent their spread by promptly removing and destroying infected plants and controlling the vectors, such as insects, that may transmit viruses.

Preventative Measures

Implement preventative measures to minimize the risk of diseases. Use disease-resistant herb varieties, rotate crops annually, and avoid overcrowding plants. Practice good garden hygiene by cleaning tools, pots, and any equipment to prevent the spread of pathogens.

CHAPTER 6: HARVESTING AND PRESERVING HERBS

Harvesting your herbs is a gratifying culmination of your gardening efforts. This chapter guides you through the best times to harvest your herbs, the art of drying and storing them for future use, and the creation of delightful herbal infusions and oils to savor the flavors and aromas of your garden.

BEST TIMES TO HARVEST

Harvesting Guidelines

Knowing when to harvest your herbs is crucial for preserving their flavor, aroma, and potency. In general, the best time to harvest herbs is in the morning after the dew has dried but before the sun is at its peak. At this time, the essential oils that contribute to flavor and fragrance are most concentrated.

Harvesting Leaves

For herbs grown for their leaves, such as basil and mint, harvest when the plants have sufficient foliage. Begin by snipping or pinching off the top leaves, and continue harvesting regularly throughout the growing season to encourage bushier growth.

Harvesting Flowers

Herbs like chamomile and lavender are prized for their flowers. Harvest flowers just as they begin to open for the best flavor and fragrance. Remove entire flower heads or individual blossoms, depending on the herb.

Harvesting Seeds

For herbs that produce seeds, such as coriander and dill, wait until the seeds are fully mature and have changed color. Harvest seed heads when they are dry, and store them in a cool, dry place to complete the drying process.

DRYING AND STORING HERBS

Air Drying

Air drying is a common traditional and effective method for preserving herbs. Bundle small bunches of herbs and hang them upside down in a dry, well-ventilated area. Ensure that the herbs are protected from direct sunlight to retain their color and essential oils.

Dehydrating

A dehydrator provides a quick and controlled method for drying herbs. Spread clean, dry herbs on dehydrator trays and follow the manufacturer's instructions. Dehydrating is particularly useful for herbs with high moisture content, like basil.

Storing Dried Herbs

Once dried, store your herbs in airtight containers to maintain freshness. Use glass jars, labeled with the herb name and harvest date. Keep containers in a cool, dark place to protect the herbs from light and temperature fluctuations.

Making Herbal Infusions and Oils

Herbal Infusions

Herbal infusions, or teas, are a delightful way to enjoy the flavors and health benefits of your herbs. Use fresh or dried herbs to create herbal teas by steeping them in hot water. Experiment with single herbs or blends to discover unique and soothing flavor combinations.

Infused Oils

Create aromatic and flavorful infused oils using your favorite herbs. Combine dried herbs with a carrier oil, such as olive oil or grapeseed oil, and let them infuse for several weeks. Strain the herbs, and you're left with a versatile infused oil perfect for culinary or skincare applications

Creating Herbal Vinegars

Enhance your culinary adventures by making herbal vinegars. Combine fresh or dried herbs with vinegar and let the mixture steep for a few weeks. Strain the herbs, and you'll have a flavorful herbal vinegar that adds a gourmet touch to salads and dishes.

CHAPTER 7: CULINARY USES OF HERBS

Herbs are nature's culinary treasures, elevating dishes with their vibrant flavors and aromatic nuances. This chapter explores the art of cooking with fresh herbs, the creation of herbal blends and infused oils, and offers beginner-friendly, herb-infused recipes to inspire your culinary journey.

Cooking with Fresh Herbs

Enhancing Flavors

Fresh herbs are a chef's secret weapon, elevating dishes with their bright flavors. Whether you're preparing savory meals or sweet treats, incorporating fresh herbs adds complexity and depth to your culinary creations.

Herb Pairing Principles

Understand the principles of herb pairing to create harmonious flavor profiles. Consider the herb's intensity, such as the boldness of rosemary or the delicacy of cilantro, and match it with complementary ingredients. Experiment with classic pairings like basil and tomatoes or mint and lamb.

Adding Herbs at the Right Time

Timing is crucial when cooking with fresh herbs. Add delicate herbs like parsley and cilantro toward the end of cooking to preserve their fresh, vibrant flavors. Hardy herbs like rosemary and thyme can withstand longer cooking times and are ideal for simmering in stews or roasting with vegetables.

Crafting Herb Blends

Experiment with crafting your own herb blends to tailor flavors to your preferences. Combine dried herbs like oregano, thyme, and rosemary for a versatile Italian blend or mix cilantro, cumin, and lime for a zesty Tex-Mex seasoning.

Infusing Oils with Herbs

Infused oils are a simple yet elegant way to incorporate herb flavors into your dishes. Experiment with different combinations, such as garlic and basil-infused olive oil for pasta or rosemary-infused oil for drizzling over roasted vegetables. These oils add a gourmet touch to your culinary creations.

Balancing Intensity

Achieve balance in your herbal blends and infused oils by considering the intensity of each herb. Some herbs, like sage and tarragon, have robust flavors and should be used sparingly, while others, like parsley and chives, offer milder notes that can be used more generously.

HERB-INFUSED RECIPES FOR BEGINNERS

1. Basil Pesto Pasta

Create a classic basil pesto by blending fresh basil, pine nuts, garlic, Parmesan cheese, and olive oil. Toss the pesto with cooked pasta for a simple and flavorful dish.

2. Rosemary Roasted Chicken

Infuse roasted chicken with the aromatic flavors of rosemary. Rub a mixture of minced rosemary, garlic, salt, and pepper onto the chicken before roasting for a delicious and aromatic main course.

3. Lemon-Thyme Vinaigrette

Whisk together fresh lemon juice, olive oil, minced thyme, Dijon mustard, and honey to create a refreshing lemon-thyme vinaigrette. Drizzle over salads for a burst of citrus herb goodness.

4. Minty Watermelon Salad

Combine cubed watermelon, feta cheese, and chopped mint for a refreshing and vibrant summer salad. The mint adds a cool and aromatic element to this delightful dish.

5. Cilantro-Lime Rice

Infuse rice with the flavors of cilantro and lime. Cook rice with minced cilantro, lime zest, and a squeeze of lime juice for a flavorful and versatile side dish.

CHAPTER 9: MEDICINAL USES OF HERBS

Beyond their culinary charm, herbs have long been revered for their medicinal properties. This chapter introduces you to the world of medicinal herbs, explores simple herbal remedies, and guides you in creating herbal teas and tinctures to harness the healing potential of nature.

INTRODUCTION TO MEDICINAL HERBS

Understanding Medicinal Properties

Medicinal herbs have been used for centuries to address various ailments and promote overall well-being. Each herb possesses unique compounds that contribute to its medicinal properties, from anti-inflammatory and antimicrobial to calming and immune-boosting.

Holistic Healing Approach

Embrace a holistic healing approach that considers the interconnectedness of the body, mind, and spirit. Medicinal herbs offer not only physical benefits but also support mental and emotional well-being. Explore the synergies between herbs and your overall health.

Respecting Traditional Knowledge:

Tap into the wealth of traditional knowledge surrounding medicinal herbs. Many cultures have long-standing herbal traditions, and learning from these practices can deepen your understanding of the therapeutic potential of herbs.

Simple Herbal Remedies

1. Calming Chamomile Infusion:

Brew a calming chamomile tea to ease stress and promote relaxation. Steep dried chamomile flowers in hot water, strain, and sweeten with honey if desired. Enjoy this soothing infusion before bedtime.

2. Echinacea Immune Boost:

Harness the immune-boosting properties of echinacea by creating a simple tincture. Combine dried echinacea root with alcohol, let it infuse for several weeks, then strain. Take a small amount daily during cold and flu seasons to support your immune system.

3. Lavender-Infused Oil for Skin:

Create a lavender-infused oil to soothe the skin and promote relaxation. Combine dried lavender flowers with a carrier oil like jojoba or almond oil and let it infuse for a few weeks. Use the infused oil for massage or as a calming addition to your skincare routine.

4. Peppermint Digestive Tea:

Brew a refreshing peppermint tea to aid digestion. Steep fresh or dried peppermint leaves in hot water, strain, and sip after meals to relieve indigestion and ease stomach discomfort.

5. Ginger Honey Cough Syrup:

Prepare a homemade cough syrup using ginger and honey. Simmer fresh ginger slices in water, strain, and mix the infused liquid with honey. Take a spoonful as needed to soothe a sore throat and calm coughs.

CREATING HERBAL TEAS AND TINCTURES

Crafting Herbal Teas

Experiment with crafting herbal teas based on your health needs and flavor preferences. Combine dried or fresh herbs like mint, lemon balm, and hibiscus to create refreshing and therapeutic blends. Adjust the ratios to achieve your desired flavor profile.

Making Herbal Tinctures

Tinctures are concentrated herbal extracts which are generally preserved in alcohol or glycerin. Create your own tinctures by combining dried herbs with alcohol, letting the mixture infuse, and then straining. Tinctures offer a convenient way to incorporate herbal remedies into your routine, and they have a longer shelf life compared to some other preparations.

Dosage and Safety Considerations

When using herbal remedies, be mindful of dosage and safety considerations. Start with little amounts and observe how your body responds. It's always advisable to consult with a healthcare professional, especially if you have pre-existing health conditions or are taking medications.

CHAPTER 9: AROMATHERAPY WITH HERBS

Aromatherapy invites you to indulge in the sensory delights of herbs, harnessing their aromatic essence for relaxation, ambiance, and well-being. This chapter introduces the extraction of essential oils from herbs, guides you in creating herbal sachets and potpourri, and offers inspiring DIY herbal aromatherapy projects.

ESSENTIAL OILS FROM HERBS

Extraction Methods

Essential oils are concentrated plant extracts that capture the aromatic compounds of herbs. Learn about various extraction methods, including steam distillation, cold pressing, and maceration.

While steam distillation is common for many herbs, some, like citrus fruits, are cold-pressed to retain their vibrant scents.

Herbs for Essential Oils

Explore herbs that are particularly suited for essential oil extraction. Lavender, rosemary, peppermint, and eucalyptus are popular choices known for their distinct fragrances and therapeutic properties. Consider cultivating these herbs or sourcing high-quality essential oils for your aromatherapy projects.

Safe Usage of Essential Oils

Exercise caution when using essential oils, as they are potent and should be diluted before direct application to the skin. Familiarize yourself with each oil's properties and consult reputable sources for recommended dilution ratios. Always perform a patch test to check for potential skin sensitivities.

Creating Herbal Sachets

Herbal sachets are delightful bundles of dried herbs that release their fragrances gradually. Make your own by combining dried herbs like lavender, rosemary, and chamomile. Place these sachets in drawers, closets, or under pillows to infuse your living spaces with calming and aromatic scents.

Crafting Potpourri Blends

Crafting potpourri allows you to blend a variety of dried herbs, flowers, and citrus peels for a customized aromatic experience. Experiment with combinations like dried rose petals, lavender buds, and cinnamon sticks. Place potpourri in decorative bowls around your home to enjoy a continuous burst of fragrance.

DIY Herbal Aromatherapy Projects

1. Relaxing Lavender Sleep Spray: Create a soothing lavender sleep spray by combining distilled water, witch hazel, and a few drops of lavender essential oil. Spritz this calming blend on your pillow before bedtime for a restful night's sleep.

2. *Invigorating Eucalyptus Shower Bombs:*

Make eucalyptus shower bombs for a revitalizing shower experience. Mix baking soda, citric acid, and eucalyptus essential oil, and shape the mixture into small bombs. Place one on the shower floor, and let the steam release the invigorating aroma.

3. *Herbal Infused Oil Diffuser:*

Craft a DIY oil diffuser using a small glass or ceramic dish. Combine carrier oil with your favorite essential oils, such as peppermint and citrus for energy or lavender and chamomile for relaxation. Place reed diffusers or bamboo skewers in the dish to disperse the fragrance throughout the room.

4. Energizing Citrus Room Spray:

Make a zesty citrus room spray by blending distilled water with citrus essential oils like orange, lemon, and grapefruit. Spritz this uplifting spray in your living spaces to create a fresh and invigorating atmosphere.

5. Rosemary and Mint Linen Sachets:

Combine dried rosemary and mint to create refreshing linen sachets. Tuck these sachets into your linen closet or dresser drawers to infuse your linens with a clean and invigorating scent.

Chapter 10: HOW TO CULTIVATE HERBS FOR TEA

Whether in a garden bed or individual pots, herbs require a minimum of six hours of sunlight daily. Well-draining soil or pots with drainage holes are essential. Outdoors, herbs often serve as companion plants along the border of a vegetable garden, but you can also create a dedicated herb corner. For indoor growth during winter, a grow light becomes necessary.

If opting for pots, ensure they are at least 10 inches in diameter. Fill each pot one-third full with Potting Mix, positioning each herb so the top of the root ball sits about an inch below the pot's rim to prevent overflow during watering.

Cover the roots with more potting soil, tamp it down firmly, and water thoroughly. A month post-planting, introduce fertilizer.

For beginners, start with a few herbs like garden sage, rosemary, and sweet mint. Explore our growing guides for more insights into cultivating herbs!

Harvesting Herbs for Tea

To ensure continuous growth and prevent flowering (and seed production), maintain a regular harvesting routine for your herbs. Opt for mornings, post-dew and before excessive heat, for the best results.

For leafy herbs like mint, lemon verbena, and thyme, avoid harvesting more than a third of the plant at once, allowing for sustained growth and repeated harvesting. For floral herbs such as roses, chamomile, or lavender, harvest when the flowers are budding, as this is when aromatic oils are most concentrated. Use sharp scissors, cutting down to the next set of leaves.

When making tea with fresh herbs, wash them gently under water, then crush the leaves with a spoon to release their oils before adding them directly to your tea. This method is particularly suitable for pleasant weather.

For drying leaves, especially during dormant months, wash and dry them gently. Arrange the leaves upside down or spread the stems on trays in a warm, airy place, turning them twice a day. Once dry and crumbly with no moisture (4 to 8 days), strip off the leaves, buds, or flowerheads and store them in airtight jars or containers. Don't forget to label them! Explore four ways to dry leaves and flowers.

Brewing Herbal Tea

Ready to brew? Consider investing in an infuser for your teacup or a teapot with built-in strainers. You can use either fresh or dried herbs, with dried herbs being more potent.

Here's a straightforward method for brewing herbal tea:

- 3 teaspoons freshly picked herbs or 1 teaspoon dried herbs
- 1 cup hot water

Instructions

Boil water, add fresh or dried herbs to an infuser in a teacup, and pour hot (not boiling) water over the herbs. Cover the cup to preserve aromas. Steep fresh herbs for up to 10 minutes, dried herbs for 4 to 6 minutes—or adjust to your preferred strength. Remove the infuser and serve.

CHAPTER 11: HERBAL TEA RECIPES

Here are 15 herbal tea recipes

You can make it from common herbs that you can find in your garden. Each recipe includes instructions and ingredients:

1. Feel Good Tea Recipe

Ideal for alleviating allergy symptoms, this tea includes echinacea and licorice known for soothing irritated throats. The bitter licorice flavor adds a refreshing kick to your morning routine.

- Boil 2 cups of water.

- Pour boiled water into a pot, add 1 tablespoon of echinacea, 1 teaspoon of dandelion root, and 1 teaspoon of licorice.

- Simmer on low heat for 15 minutes.

- Strain the tea through a basket or small metal strainer into a mug or tea cup.

- Add a heaping teaspoon of honey to taste.

2. Minty Tea Recipe

With an abundance of mint from your garden, try this minty tea recipe featuring peppermint leaves, catnip leaves, rose petals, and lemon verbena leaves.

- Dry the herbs as described earlier.

- Pour boiling water over the herbs, cover, and steep for 3 to 5 minutes.

- Sweeten with honey if desired.

For those herbs and more, check your local health food store or start your own herbal garden!

3. Minty Fresh Tea

Ingredients:

- Fresh mint leaves

- Boiling water

- Honey (optional)

Instructions:

1. Place a handful of fresh mint leaves in a teapot.

2. Pour boiling water over the leaves.

3. Let it steep for 5-7 minutes.

4. Strain and sweeten with honey if desired.

4. . Lemon Balm Delight

Ingredients:

- Lemon balm leaves

- Lemon slices

- Boiling water

- Agave syrup (optional)

Instructions:

1. Combine lemon balm leaves and lemon slices in a teapot.

2. Pour boiling water over the mixture.

3. Steep for 7-10 minutes.

4. Strain and sweeten with agave syrup if desired.

5. Rosemary Citrus Infusion

Ingredients:

- Fresh rosemary sprigs

- Orange peel

- Boiling water

- Maple syrup (optional)

Instructions:

1. Add fresh rosemary sprigs and orange peel to a teapot.

2. Pour boiling water over the herbs.

3. Steep for 8-10 minutes.

4. Strain and sweeten with maple syrup if desired.

6. Lavender Chamomile Blend

Ingredients:

- Lavender flowers

- Chamomile flowers

- Boiling water

- Lemon wedge (optional)

Instructions:

1. Combine lavender and chamomile flowers in a teapot.

2. Pour boiling water over the blend.

3. Steep for 5-7 minutes.

4. Strain and add a lemon wedge if desired.

7. Basil Ginger Elixir

Ingredients:

- Fresh basil leaves

- Ginger slices

- Boiling water

- Raw honey (optional.

Instructions:

1. Place fresh basil leaves and ginger slices in a teapot.

2. Pour boiling water over the herbs.

3. Steep for 7-10 minutes.

4. Strain and sweeten with raw honey if desired.

8. Thyme and Lemon Zest Tea

Ingredients:

- Fresh thyme sprigs

- Lemon zest

- Boiling water

- Agave nectar (optional)

Instructions:

1. Add fresh thyme sprigs and lemon zest to a teapot.

2. Pour boiling water over the mixture.

3. Steep for 6-8 minutes.

4. Strain and sweeten with agave nectar if desired.

9. Sage and Blackberry Bliss

Ingredients:

- Fresh sage leaves

- Blackberries

- Boiling water

- Stevia leaves (optional)

Instructions:

1. Combine fresh sage leaves and blackberries in a teapot.

2. Pour boiling water over the blend.

3. Steep for 8-10 minutes.

4. Strain and sweeten with stevia leaves if desired.

10. Cinnamon Rose Hibiscus Tea

Ingredients:

- Cinnamon sticks

- Dried rose petals

- Hibiscus flowers

- Boiling water

- Brown sugar (optional)

Instructions:

1. Add cinnamon sticks, dried rose petals, and hibiscus flowers to a teapot.

2. Pour boiling water over the herbs.

3. Steep for 7-9 minutes.

4. Strain and sweeten with brown sugar if desired.

11. Lemon Verbena and Mint Fusion

Ingredients:

- Lemon verbena leaves

- Fresh mint leaves

- Boiling water

- Agave syrup (optional)

Instructions:

1. Combine lemon verbena leaves and fresh mint leaves in a teapot.

2. Pour boiling water over the mixture.

3. Steep for 5-7 minutes.

4. Strain and sweeten with agave syrup if desired.

12. Dandelion Root Detox Tea

Ingredients:

- Dandelion root (roasted)

- Burdock root

- Boiling water

- Raw honey (optional)

Instructions:

1. Add roasted dandelion root and burdock root to a teapot.

2. Pour boiling water over the roots.

3. Steep for 10-12 minutes.

4. Strain and sweeten with raw honey if desired.

13. Lemon Thyme Serenity

Ingredients:

- Lemon thyme leaves

- Lemon slices

- Boiling water

- Maple syrup (optional)

Instructions:

1. Place lemon thyme leaves and lemon slices in a teapot.

2. Pour boiling water over the herbs.

3. Steep for 6-8 minutes.

4. Strain and sweeten with maple syrup if desired.

14. Parsley and Lemon Verbena Refresher

Ingredients:

- Fresh parsley leaves

- Lemon verbena leaves

- Boiling water

- Stevia leaves (optional)

Instructions:

1. Combine fresh parsley leaves and lemon verbena leaves in a teapot.

2. Pour boiling water over the mixture.

3. Steep for 7-9 minutes.

4. Strain and sweeten with stevia leaves if desired.

15. Fennel and Peppermint Soother

Ingredients:

- Fennel seeds

- Fresh peppermint leaves

- Boiling water

- Raw honey (optional)

Instructions:

1. Add fennel seeds and fresh peppermint leaves to a teapot.

2. Pour boiling water over the herbs.

3. Steep for 8-10 minutes.

4. Strain and sweeten with raw honey if desired.

Feel free to adjust the quantities of herbs and sweeteners according to your taste preferences. *Enjoy your herbal tea journey!*

CHAPTER 12: TOP 21 PLANTS FOR YOUR HERBAL TEA GARDEN

Indulge in the joy of growing an herbal tea garden if you're a plant enthusiast who loves sipping on comforting beverages. Join farmer Briana Yablonski as she unveils 21 of the finest plants tailored for your herbal tea haven.

When people envision edible gardens, thoughts often gravitate towards vegetables like tomatoes or herbs like dill and parsley. However, the realm of herbal teas opens up a diverse array of plants to cultivate. Whether craving a revitalizing mint infusion or a zesty citrus blend, your garden holds the key.

1. Lemon Balm

- Botanical Name: Melissa officinalis
- Sunlight Needs: Full sun to partial shade
- Height: 3 feet
- Hardiness Zones: 4–9

Lemon balm, a fragrant perennial herb, boasts tender green leaves with a citrus essence. Perfect for tea or as a delightful bouquet filler, this hardy and easily grown herb suits both beginners and seasoned gardeners. Plant it in well-draining soil, ensuring at least six hours of sunlight for a happy, thriving lemon balm. Exercise caution, though, as it tends to spread—consider containing it near a rock border or in a pot.

2. German Chamomile

- Botanical Name: Matricaria recutita
- Sun Requirements: Full sun
- Height: 1–2 feet
- Hardiness Zones: 3–10

Renowned for its calming benefits, German chamomile provides a remarkable taste for fresh chamomile tea, surpassing traditional tea bags. As an annual plant with small daisy-like flowers, harvesting mature flowers stimulates continuous blooming throughout the summer. Though an annual, German chamomile's reseeding capability may surprise you. For an attractive garden, plant multiple clumps or scatter seedlings to entice pollinators. Seedlings prefer moist soil, while mature plants exhibit tolerance to moderate drought.

3. Lemongrass

- Botanical Name: Cymbopogon citratus
- Sun Requirements: Full sun
- Height: 4–5 feet
- Hardiness Zones: 4–9

Not just a staple in curry paste and Thai soups, lemongrass contributes a vibrant, citrusy flavor to herbal teas. Utilize the entire stem and leaves for tea, and plant it outdoors after the risk of frost subsides. Set seedlings in well-drained, sunny locations, keeping the soil consistently moist. While lemongrass takes several months to develop thick stems, you can harvest leaves throughout spring and summer. Come frost, the plants may die, but you can dig them up and store them indoors for replanting in the following spring.

4. Ginger

- Botanical Name: Zingiber officinale
- Sun Requirements: Full sun to partial shade
- Height: 3–4 feet
- Hardiness Zones: 4–9

Experience the excitement of growing baby ginger, with tender, spicy rhizomes and lush green leaves as the ultimate reward. Plant ginger outdoors once temperatures consistently stay above 50°F, and provide ample moisture and nutrients. Harvest portions of ginger rhizomes in the fall, appreciating their tenderness compared to store-bought counterparts. Use baby ginger promptly or freeze for future use.

5. Bronze Fennel

- Botanical Name: Foeniculum vulgare 'Bronze'
- Sun Requirements: Full sun
- Height: 1–3 feet
- Hardiness Zones: 3–9

Bronze fennel, offering an anise flavor akin to culinary fennel, showcases red, feathery fronds rather than a bulb. A perennial herb, it enhances the sweetness of herbal tea, either standalone or blended with other herbs. With its yellow, umbel-shaped flowers, bronze fennel adds not only flavor but also visual appeal to your teas and garnishes.

6. Peppermint

Peppermint, a favored choice for herbal tea, offers a refreshing and crisp mint flavor suitable for both fresh and dried leaves.

-Botanical Name: Mentha x piperita

- Sun Requirements: Full sun to partial shade

- Height: 1–3 feet

- Hardiness Zones: 3–8

Peppermint, thriving in at least six hours of daily sun and well-draining soil, is an easy-to-grow plant. While it can withstand some drought, moderately moist soil is preferable.

Caution is advised when planting it directly in the garden, as it tends to spread. To contain it, consider a solid-bordered area like a raised bed or keep it in a pot. As a perennial, peppermint returns for multiple years, and propagation through division or stem cuttings facilitates expansion to new garden areas.

7. Catnip

Catnip, known for its appeal to cats, doubles as an excellent addition to herbal tea gardens, potentially offering relaxing properties when steeped.

- Botanical Name: Nepeta cataria

- Sun Requirements: Full sun

- Height: 2–3 feet

- Hardiness Zones: 3–7

Catnip, a perennial growing in small clumps, thrives in well-draining soil and full sun. While recognized for its feline attraction, the leaves or flowers steeped in water may produce a tea with purported relaxing effects on humans. Research on its impact on human health is limited, but caution is advised as it can spread aggressively.

8. Anise Hyssop

Anise hyssop, part of the mint family, is a short-lived perennial with an anise-like fragrance, creating a subtly sweet tea with a mild black licorice flavor.

- Botanical Name: Agastache foeniculum
- Sun Requirements: Full sun
- Height: 2–4 feet

- Hardiness Zones: 4–9

This aromatic plant, with a potential height and width of up to four feet, thrives in garden spaces with good airflow. A member of the mint family, anise hyssop's fragrant leaves, and flowers contribute to an herbal tea with a delightful licorice flavor. Apart from its culinary appeal, it serves as a pollinator magnet, attracting bees, butterflies, and hoverflies with its purple flower spikes.

9. Holy Basil

Holy basil, also known as tulsi, belongs to the basil genus, offering potential health benefits and adaptogenic properties in Ayurvedic and Chinese medicine.

- Botanical Name: Ocimum sanctum

- Sun Requirements: Full sun

- Height: 2 feet

- Hardiness Zones: 10–11

As a close relative to true basil, holy basil or tulsi is valued not only for its use in Thai cuisine but also for potential stress-adaptation properties. While it grows perennially in warmer U.S. regions, it behaves as an annual in most areas. Plant tulsi in well-drained soil and full sun for optimal growth.

10. Rosemary

Rosemary, a drought-tolerant perennial shrub, thrives in dry, well-drained areas, making it an ideal choice for herbal tea gardens.

- Botanical Name: Salvia rosmarinus

- Sun Requirements: Full sun

- Height: 2–5 feet

- Hardiness Zones: 7–11

Ideal for arid conditions, rosemary, a low-maintenance shrub, dislikes oversaturated soil. In colder regions, it dies back but can be moved indoors during winter. Regular pruning by clipping the tips enhances fragrance for tea and maintains the plant's shape. Aim for annual pruning, removing about one-third of the foliage in late spring and fall.

11. Rose

Roses, typically admired for their garden beauty, offer more than just visual appeal—they can be used to craft antioxidant-rich herbal tea from both their petals and rose hips.

- Botanical Name: Rosa spp.
- Sunlight Needs: Full sunlight to partial shade
- Height: 2–12 feet
- Hardiness Zones: 3–10

Beyond their ornamental value, roses contribute to herbal tea with a fruity and floral flavor derived from both their petals and rose hips. While any rose type can be used, certain species, like wild or native roses (e.g., swamp rose, Carolina rose, Virginia rose), tend to yield more rose hips. To harvest both petals and hips, leave some flowers on the plant for them to develop into rose hips.

12. Purple Coneflower

Purple coneflower, known for its antioxidant-rich roots, imparts an earthy-floral flavor to herbal tea.

- Botanical Name: Echinacea purpurea
- Sun Requirements: Full sun
- Height: 2–3 feet
- Hardiness Zones: 4–9

The roots of purple coneflower have long been utilized to create herbal tea rich in antioxidants. Flourishing in clumps with purple and pink flowers, this perennial attracts butterflies, bees, and other pollinators. Adaptable to poor soil and drought, purple coneflower is a low-maintenance choice for herbal tea gardens.

13. Lemon Verbena

Lemon verbena, a fragrant perennial shrub, yields a revitalizing tea with its citrusy leaves.

- Botanical Name: Aloysia citriodora
- Sun Requirements: Full sun
- Height: 3–8 feet
- Hardiness Zones: 8–11

Lemon verbena, a tender perennial, produces bright green leaves with a citrusy fragrance. Brewing these leaves in hot water results in a refreshing tea, and combining lemon verbena with less palatable herbs enhances the overall flavor. While it may not survive colder regions, container gardening allows for winter relocation. With a preference for full sun and consistent moisture, lemon verbena maintains its appeal without aggressive spreading.

14. White Horehound

White horehound, with a slightly bitter, menthol-like flavor, is recognized for its use in soothing teas.

- Botanical Name: Marrubium vulgare
- Sun Requirements: Full sun
- Height: 2–3 feet
- Hardiness Zones: 3–9

Known for its slightly bitter taste resembling menthol, white horehound has historical use in throat-soothing remedies. A member of the mint family, it may spread rapidly, warranting close monitoring or container planting to control its growth. While seeds take time to germinate, once past the seedling stage, the plant proves easy to cultivate with well-draining soil and moderate moisture.

15. Common Chicory

Chicory, recognized for its periwinkle flowers, presents a robust taproot suitable for herbal tea.

- Botanical Name: Cichorium intybus
- Sun Requirements: Full sun
- Height: 3–5 feet
- Hardiness Zones: 3–9

Known for its periwinkle flowers, chicory, a perennial, offers a robust taproot ideal for herbal tea. Thriving in loose, well-drained soil, chicory exhibits rapid vegetative growth in the first year, delaying flowering until the second year. Although roots can be harvested at any time, waiting for mature plants ensures larger yields. Notably, roasted chicory root serves as a coffee substitute with a mildly bitter flavor.

16. English Lavender

English lavender, an aromatic shrub, imparts a subtly sweet, floral essence to tea, enhancing both flavor and fragrance.

- Botanical Name: Lavandula angustifolia
- Sun Requirements: Full sun
- Height: 2 feet
- Hardiness Zones: 5–10

Amidst the diverse lavender species, English lavender stands out for its subtly sweet and floral aroma, enriching teas, syrups, and baked goods.

Flourishing in a dry, sunny environment akin to its Mediterranean origin, it thrives in well-drained soil. Both fragrant sage-colored leaves and bright purple flowers contribute to tea-making, with dried parts retaining flavor for future use.

17. Purple Passionflower

Purple passionflower, a vining plant, is renowned for its intricate purple flowers and tendrils, often used in herbal teas.
- Botanical Name: Passiflora incarnata
- Sunlight Needs: Full sunlight to partial shade
- Height: 10–25 feet
- Hardiness Zones: 5–9

A vining, flowering plant, purple passion flower captivates with intricate, large purple flowers and delicious passionfruit. Although typically cultivated for its fruit, the leaves and tendrils find application in herbal tea. Versatile in growth, it thrives on support structures or trails through gardens, returning yearly in warm zones. Winter sees above-ground portions dying back, only to resurge in spring.

18. Valerian

Valerian, recognized for its calming effects, is a hardy perennial suitable for herbal tea, especially when balanced with complementary flavors.

- Botanical Name: Valeriana officinalis
- Sun Requirements: Full sun

- Height: 3–5 feet

- Hardiness Zones: 3–9

Valerian, popular for its relaxation and insomnia-alleviating properties, can be easily grown at home. Thriving in various soil types, it prefers full sun conditions with well-draining soil. Harvesting valerian roots in spring or fall, followed by a careful drying process, ensures optimal use. Due to its acquired taste, blending with appealing flavors like ginger or lemon verbena enhances its palatability.

19. Roselle

Hibiscus sabdariffa, known as Roselle or Jamaican Sorrel, produces vibrant red calyces for a tart herbal tea.

- Botanical Name: Hibiscus sabdariffa
- Sun Requirements: Full sun
- Height: 5–7 feet
- Hardiness Zones: 8–11

Hibiscus sabdariffa, commonly called Roselle or Jamaican Sorrel, distinguishes itself with bright red calyces ideal for crafting a tart herbal tea. While native to West Africa and thriving in warm winters, potted cultivation extends its reach. Abundant sun and moisture support the growth of cream-colored summer flowers and fall's red calyces, ready for immediate use or subsequent drying.

20. Lemon Thyme

Lemon thyme, with its citrusy flavor, adds a delightful taste to teas and a pleasant fragrance to the garden.

- Botanical Name: Thymus citriodorus
- Sun Requirements: Full sun
- Height: 6–12 inches
- Hardiness Zones: 5–9

Lemon thyme, belonging to the low-growing and drought-tolerant thyme family, elevates herbal teas with a citrusy essence. Ideal for rock gardens or between paving stones, it thrives with ample sunlight. Regular trimming promotes new

21. Calendula

Calendula, scientifically known as Calendula officinalis, is an annual herb boasting lance-shaped, bright green leaves and vibrant, daisy-like flowers in shades of bright orange and yellow. These distinctive double-petal flowers are held on sturdy stems, creating a visually striking display.

- Botanical Name: Calendula officinalis
- Sun Requirements: Full sun
- Height: 1–2 feet
- Hardiness Zones: 3–11

Calendula stands out as a versatile annual plant, showcasing a profusion of daisy-like flowers that are ideal for herbal tea. The plants have a unique C-shaped seed, and their blooms feature a double-petal structure. To ensure continuous flowering for three to four months, diligent deadheading is recommended.

CULTIVATION

To cultivate calendula, sow the distinctive C-shaped seeds in your garden after the threat of frost has passed. Optimal results are achieved in well-draining soil with full sun exposure. The seeds quickly germinate, and within a couple of months, the plants begin producing a delightful array of blooms.

VARIETIES

Calendula offers a spectrum of flower colors, providing options for personal preference. Varieties like 'Resin Calendula' boast bright orange blooms, while 'Zeolights Calendula' presents flowers in shades of pink and salmon.

CHAPTER 13: TROUBLESHOOTING COMMON ISSUES

Embarking on an herb gardening journey is not without its challenges. This chapter provides valuable insights into addressing common gardening challenges and tackles herb-specific issues to ensure your garden thrives.

ADDRESSING COMMON GARDENING CHALLENGES

1. Soil Quality and Drainage

Challenge: Poor soil quality or inadequate drainage can hinder herb growth.

Solution: Test your soil, amend it with organic matter, and ensure proper drainage by adding materials like perlite or sand.

Pests and Diseases

Challenge: Insects and diseases can impact herb health.

Solution: Implement pest prevention strategies, practice companion planting, and promptly address any signs of diseases with appropriate treatments.

Overwatering and Underwatering

Challenge: Inconsistent watering practices can lead to stressed plants.

Solution: Establish a regular watering schedule, adjust based on weather conditions, and use well-draining soil to prevent waterlogged roots.

Sunlight Issues

Challenge: Insufficient or excessive sunlight can affect herb growth.

Solution: Position your herb garden in a location that receives the appropriate amount of sunlight based on the needs of your specific herbs.

TROUBLESHOOTING HERB-SPECIFIC ISSUES

1. Basil Yellowing Leaves

Issue: Yellowing basil leaves may indicate overwatering or nutrient deficiency.

Solution: Adjust your watering routine, ensure proper drainage, and feed your basil with a balanced fertilizer.

Rosemary Dieback Issue

Rosemary plants experiencing dieback may be affected by fungal diseases or poor soil drainage.

Solution: Improve soil drainage, avoid overhead watering, and prune affected branches to encourage new growth.

Mint Overgrowth Issue

Mint can be invasive and overtake other plants in the garden.

Solution: Plant mint in containers to control its spread, or designate a separate area for it to prevent it from dominating the garden.

Thyme Drying Out Issue

Thyme plants drying out may be a result of insufficient water or overly compacted soil.

Solution: Water thyme consistently, and ensure the soil is well-draining. Addition of organic matter to improve soil structure.

CONCLUSION

In conclusion, the appeal of calendula extends beyond its aesthetic qualities, making it a versatile addition to various garden settings, including cut flower beds, pollinator gardens, and herbal tea gardens.

The process of growing calendula is straightforward, involving considerations such as sun exposure, well-draining soil, and regular deadheading.

With its diverse flower colors, calendula adds a vibrant touch to any garden, contributing to the overall charm of an herbal tea garden.

As you embark on this botanical journey, the abundance of plant choices may pose the delightful challenge of selecting the perfect herbs based on your flavor preferences, growing zone, and garden size.

Embrace the journey, savor the flavors, and revel in the aromatic beauty of your herb garden.

Happy gardening!